First Steps
to living with
Dementia

Dr Simon Atkins

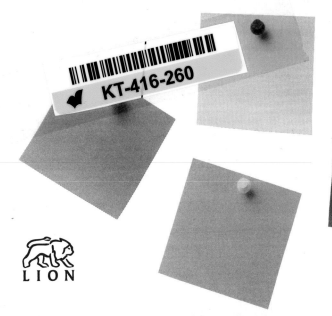

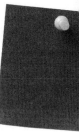

KT-416-260

LION

Dedicated to the memory of my grandmother
Hilda Taylor and my uncle George Hardyman.

*With special thanks to Ruth Clarke for all her
help while preparing the manuscript and to my wife
Nikki for her support while I was researching and
writing it.*

Text copyright © 2013 Simon Atkins
This edition copyright © 2013 Lion Hudson

The right of Simon Atkins to be identified as the author of this work has been
asserted by him in accordance with the Copyright, Designs and Patents Act 1988.

Published by Lion Books
an imprint of
Lion Hudson plc
Wilkinson House, Jordan Hill Road,
Oxford OX2 8DR, England
www.lionhudson.com/lion

ISBN 978 0 7459 5556 8
e-ISBN 978 0 7459 5721 0

First edition 2013

Acknowledgments
p. 12: Figures from the Alzheimer's Society website reprinted by permission of
Alzheimer's Society UK, 2012: alzheimers.org.uk/infographic.
p. 73: *The Poems* by Dylan Thomas © Dylan Thomas. Reprinted by permission of
David Higham Associates and New Direction.
p. 59: "My mother was back, the lights were on" by Oliver James, *The Guardian*,
2nd August 2008. Reprinted by permission of Guardian New & Media Ltd.

Diagram p. 86 © Sam Atkins, redrawn by Jonathan Roberts

Cover and p. 3 image © Uyen Le/iStockphoto.com

A catalogue record for this book is available from the British Library

Printed and bound in the UK, January 2015, LH26

Contents

Foreword

A short while ago I was away for the weekend and found myself sitting around the supper table with six people I had only just met. Inevitably perhaps, the conversation started with what each of us did. The first to respond said that she was actually having a much-needed break, courtesy of the rest of her family, since she was a full-time carer for her mother, who had Alzheimer's disease. Immediately, another interjected that she too had a mother in the same condition. The topic of the evening immediately switched from careers to dementia...

As we talked through the histories of what had happened, the personal anecdotes, and the more general issues involved, from basic neuroscience to practical needs, it became clear that these two women were desperate for information. No one, they said, had really explained things to them; no one had given them the full picture. Already, as the evening progressed, they were feeling more positive. Of course, they realized that there was currently no cure for dementia, but just understanding more was, for them, a morale boost.

Life sometimes delivers weird coincidences. Amazingly, that very weekend I had packed in my luggage the manuscript of this book, sent to me by Simon Atkins. It struck me that this was just the kind of thing that was evidently needed and currently not readily available in a simple, concise guide. The very questions raised at our dinner were, I'm sure, typical of those in the minds of many who are now having their worlds tilted by the devastating realization of dementia. Dr Atkins' book is remarkable in that it covers the whole gamut of issues, from a basic introduction to the brain through to advice on legal and financial help, and it does so in a concise and lucid, highly readable way. Above all, here is a compassionate overview from someone who knows what it is like to feel that someone you love is slipping away. Although it offers no magic bullet, no prospect of some easy snake-oil answer, it is an honest and clear account of the current state of play in understanding dementia. And, as I found with my supper companions, understanding is the first step forward.

Baroness Susan Greenfield
Neuroscientist at the University of Oxford
researching into Alzheimer's disease

Introduction

Every seven seconds someone in the world is diagnosed with dementia.

No, that's not a typo. You can even rub your eyes and re-read it if you like, but the statistic won't have changed. In fact, by the time you've done all that, there will already have been a new case diagnosed somewhere else.

But perhaps it is worth reading again, because it's quite a shocking statistic that may take a while to sink in. And what it means is that by the time you've watched an average-length movie or your favourite team playing ninety minutes of football, there are almost another 850 people on the planet who've been given that diagnosis.

To bring it closer to home, it may only be a matter of time before you or I are given that news ourselves. And, without a shadow of a doubt, it guarantees that someone we know and love will one day be told that they have dementia.

And we are only talking about those people who are actually being given a diagnosis. There is concern that family doctors like me are only picking up half the cases in our practices that we should be. This could be the tip of a very much larger, and scarier, iceberg.

So, what do we mean by dementia?

We have all had what's laughingly called a "senior moment". We forget where we left our car keys, for example, and then, after frantically turning the house upside down, find they were in our pocket all along. Or we bump into an old neighbour for the first time in ages and, despite having nattered to them over the garden fence for more than a decade, find it impossible to think of a name to fit their familiar face.

Then there are the times when we get in a muddle and pour tea into the sugar bowl, or forget to take the Yorkshire puddings out of the oven with the roast, only to be reminded of them five minutes later by the whiff of burning batter.

And finally there are those awful, chilling moments when we are enjoying a latte and a chat with friends and it suddenly dawns on us that we should have been at the dentist across town ten minutes ago or, worse still, we've missed school pick-up time and our six-year-old will by now be a snivelling wreck in their teacher's arms.

I could go on listing examples because it's very common, and thankfully completely normal, for all of us to forget even very familiar and important things every now and again. But when does this forgetfulness become pathological? How many senior moments do you need to have before it becomes worrying? When does serial absent-mindedness stop being a quirky part of someone's personality and signify the early signs of dementia? And how do we find out?

Whether you are concerned for yourself or a loved one, or whether the diagnosis has already been made, that's where this little book comes in. It will look at what dementia is, and what it isn't, and discuss the four main different types (as well as some of the rarer ones). It will highlight the common symptoms to be aware of and how to go about confirming the diagnosis, with sections giving details of the common tests used by doctors and psychologists to investigate things further.

Treatments will also be covered, including those offered by both the medical profession and complementary therapists, paying particular attention to the ways in which relatives and carers can help. And finally we will look at the long-term outlook, how the condition is likely to progress, and what can be done to minimize distress as it does.

Thankfully, it's not all gloom and doom. Advances in drug treatments, social and psychological therapies, and greater awareness are already helping people with dementia to maintain a better quality of life than would have been possible even a decade ago. But with at least another dozen people being diagnosed since you opened this book, there's a real urgency for all of us to be more aware of this disabling and, so far, incurable condition.

1

What is dementia?

Dementia is caused by a number of different illnesses which each lead to progressive and irreversible damage to the brain. Symptoms caused by this damage can include loss of memory, confusion, disorientation, problems with language and judgment, lack of insight, mood changes, hallucinations and delusions, and, as a result, the gradual loss of the ability to carry out even the most basic tasks of daily living.

It is a condition of adults that can affect both men and women and becomes more common with increasing age, although 2 per cent of those diagnosed are younger than 65. Once picked up, symptoms can be stable for up to five years and the average survival rate is around ten years (although this depends on age at diagnosis). This reduced survival compared to the rest of the population is likely to be due to the incapacity caused by dementia, which increases the risk of falls as well as susceptibility to picking up infections such as pneumonia.

Dementia by numbers

800,000	The number of people with dementia in the UK.
1.7 million	The number of people with dementia in the UK by 2051.
1 in 3	The number of people over the age of 65 who will develop dementia.
62%	The proportion of people with dementia that is caused by Alzheimer's disease.
£23 billion	The cost of dementia to the UK.
£8 billion	The value to the UK of work done by carers.

Source: Alzheimer's Society, 2012

Mythbuster

All old people get dementia.
Dementia is not a normal part of ageing, and although one in three people over 65 will develop it, that means that a massive two-thirds of the elderly population will not.

The most common cause of dementia is Alzheimer's disease, with vascular disease, frontal lobe dementia (or Pick's disease), and Lewy body disease being the next most common causes. Age distribution for causes of dementia is shaped like a funnel – wide at the top and much narrower at the bottom – because in younger people any of the diseases can be responsible, whereas in the over-75s it's almost exclusively down to Alzheimer's.

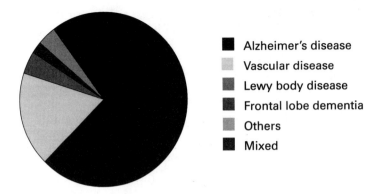

Alzheimer's disease
Vascular disease
Lewy body disease
Frontal lobe dementia
Others
Mixed

In order to understand what goes wrong inside our brain when we develop any type of dementia, it can help to have some idea about how the brain works when it's doing its job properly. Go to Appendix A to find out more.

Alzheimer's disease

This is the most frequent cause of dementia, which, because we are all living longer, is predicted to affect over 80 million people across the globe by 2040. That's a whopping four times the number affected now.

First described by a German doctor called Alois Alzheimer in 1906, it is a physical disease that causes protein plaques and tangles to form in brain cells. These cause damage to the cells, which stops them working properly and eventually leads to cell death. As time goes on, the disease spreads to more and more parts of the brain, making the symptoms worse.

There is no single cause of Alzheimer's disease, but there is thought to be an inherited (genetic) risk, with lifestyle factors such as smoking and poor diet also being significant risk factors. By far the biggest risk factor is age, with 99 per cent of cases occurring in people over the age of 65.

Vascular dementia

This is the second most common form of dementia. It is not in itself a single disease but is caused by damage to small blood vessels in the brain either by atherosclerosis (furring of the arteries) or by small haemorrhages. It can also be caused by the effects of poor circulation due to heart failure.

Strokes are the biggest culprits, with 25 per cent of people who have had a stroke developing symptoms of dementia within one year.

The risk factors for this type of dementia are diabetes, high blood pressure, raised cholesterol levels, smoking, poor diet, and lack of exercise.

Mixed dementia

Given that, like Alzheimer's disease, the risk of vascular dementia goes up with age, it's very common to find people whose dementia symptoms are caused by a mixture of the two conditions.

Lewy body disease

This disease, like Alzheimer's, bears the name of the doctor who first described it. In this case it was Frederic Lewy, working in 1912, who first noted abnormal, spherical protein deposits in the midbrain and cortex. These deposits are also found in the midbrains of people who have Parkinson's disease and so, in Lewy body disease, sufferers not only have the symptoms of dementia but tend to have Parkinson's symptoms too (see Chapter 2 for more detail on symptoms).

Alongside the Lewy body proteins, the brains of people with this type of dementia are also often damaged by the presence of plaques and tangles.

The cause of this condition is still a mystery despite a lot of research.

Frontal lobe dementia

This type of dementia was originally known as Pick's disease after Arnold Pick, a psychiatrist working in Prague, who first recorded it in 1892. It has since been rebranded as frontal lobe or frontotemporal dementia to include other conditions, such as motor neurone disease, which can cause dementia affecting these areas of the brain (the frontal and temporal lobes).

The cause is again unknown and its symptoms are mentioned in Chapter 2.

Other causes

A large number of other diseases can cause damage to the brain and lead to symptoms of dementia. Some of these are conditions that affect the brain directly, but disturbances in levels of the body's chemicals and hormones, along with various infections, can also cause dementia-like symptoms. Many of these are treatable (urinary infections, for example) and not chronic and progressive illnesses like the diseases we've just looked at.

➤ Neurological causes

Parkinson's disease (PD)

People with this condition have a higher risk than average of developing dementia and make up 2 per cent of all people suffering with dementia. People with PD-related dementia have similar symptoms to those with Lewy body disease, and there may be a link between the two. In addition to the common symptoms of dementia, they suffer with visual hallucinations and may also have mood swings and episodes of irritability. Unfortunately, some of the drugs used to treat their PD may make their dementia symptoms worse.

Multiple sclerosis (MS)

It's reckoned that a high percentage of people with MS have some sort of cognitive problems. They are particularly susceptible if their MS affects the cortex of the brain.

Normal pressure hydrocephalus (NPH)

It can be difficult to tell the difference between NPH, Alzheimer's, and PD because the symptoms overlap. In NPH there is an accumulation of fluid in the brain which causes the ventricles to enlarge. This stretches the brain tissue, causing the symptoms of dementia, walking difficulties, and incontinence of urine. It affects people over the age of 55 and has to be treated by brain surgeons, who put a shunt into the brain to drain the fluid.

Creutzfeldt–Jakob disease (CJD)

This rare brain disease has four types, the best known of which is vCJD, which was once thought to be linked to so-called "Mad Cow" disease. Although no link was proven, it is believed that this type of CJD may be contagious, whereas the others are more commonly either sporadic or genetic. Dementia is only one small feature of this awful disease, which causes multiple neurological symptoms such as unsteadiness, slurred speech, loss of bladder control, and blindness.

Huntington's disease
This is a hereditary disease caused by a faulty gene on chromosome 4. If one parent has the disease, then there is a fifty-fifty chance of a child inheriting it. Symptoms begin in middle age (30–50 years) and progress relentlessly until death. Alongside dementia, symptoms include loss of movement control and mood changes. Huntington's disease eventually leads to the complete inability of sufferers to look after themselves.

➤ Hormonal and nutritional causes

Addison's disease and Cushing's disease
In these diseases there is either too little (Addison's) or too much (Cushing's) of a hormone called cortisol. This leads to imbalances in mineral levels in the blood, such as sodium and potassium, which, among other things, can cause mental confusion. Treatment of the underlying triggers can help alleviate these symptoms.

Diabetes
Low blood-sugar levels can cause confusion and disorientation similar to that seen in dementia. Correcting the level of sugar by simply giving some chocolate can

solve the problem in the short term. It can be prevented by good diabetes control.

Thyroid disease

The thyroid gland produces hormones that help control metabolism. An over- or underactive thyroid gland can cause symptoms of confusion and upset thought processes because of the abnormal levels of these hormones. Again, treating the thyroid disease will cure these symptoms.

Hyperparathyroidism

The parathyroid glands make a hormone that controls the body's levels of calcium, phosphorus, and vitamin D. Overproduction of the hormone will put the blood level of calcium up too high. This can cause changes in personality, altered levels of consciousness, disorientation, and even coma.

Vitamin B12 deficiency

One of the jobs of this B vitamin is to ensure normal function of the nervous system. It is found in various foods and absorbed through the digestive system. Unfortunately, some people are unable to absorb it and as a result can end up with damage to nerves in their arms, legs, and brain. Injections are available to sort out the deficiency, but if it has taken a while to diagnose, it may be too late to reverse damage that's already been done.

Cirrhosis

Damage to liver cells from either alcohol or infections, such as viral hepatitis, will stop the liver from performing its usual functions, which include the removal of toxic waste products from the blood stream. If these toxins build up, they can cause damage to brain cells, causing confusion, forgetfulness, changes in personality, and inappropriate behaviour, which together are called "encephalopathy". These symptoms can sometimes be reversed by treating the liver damage, but in severe cases encephalopathy can be fatal.

➤ Alcohol-related causes

Korsakoff's syndrome
This condition occurs mostly in alcoholics. Excess alcohol consumption reduces the absorption of a vitamin called thiamine, which is needed for brain cells to work normally. Lack of this vitamin causes memory problems and a change in personality. It can be treated by stopping drinking and by taking thiamine and other vitamin supplements.

Infectious causes
Infections that directly affect the brain, such as meningitis and encephalitis, can cause confusion and altered mental states. But, especially in the elderly, infections of the urinary tract or even the chest can have the same effect.

 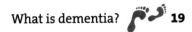

2

Symptoms of dementia

Identifying the symptoms of dementia as early as possible is crucial because it means that sufferers can get the help they need quickly, and carers and relatives can start planning for their loved ones' likely future needs. But at the same time we have to be careful that we don't look so hard for these symptoms that we see dementia behind every senior moment and whisk Granddad off to the nearest nursing home after a couple of lapses of memory.

Types of symptoms

There are three main categories of symptoms that are relevant to all of the main different types of dementia.
   These are:

• *cognitive (thought processing) problems* – affecting people's memory, their ability to learn new things, their understanding, and problem-solving ability

- *emotional problems* – affecting mood (causing depression and irritability) and social interaction with other people

- *functional problems* – affecting ability to carry out normal daily activities such as washing, dressing, and cooking meals.

Stages of symptom development

Dementia is a progressive condition, with symptoms becoming more severe as time goes on. The development of these symptoms can be split into three stages:

- early or mild dementia

- moderate dementia

- severe dementia.

The rate at which someone proceeds through these stages will differ, depending on the underlying causes of their dementia and the stage at which their dementia is diagnosed. It can also be slowed down by their educational background, with those who stayed in education longer being able to compensate better for the symptoms of dementia.

Early dementia can, however, take many years to identify, as the mild symptoms can be put down to normal ageing or depression and could simply be a form of mild cognitive impairment (see later). In moderate dementia there is little doubt that someone has it, as they will invariably need supervision to carry out most tasks, and by the time dementia is severe, the person has lost the ability to live independently at all and needs constant care.

The different types of dementia also seem to progress at different rates, with the frontotemporal type being much more rapid than either Alzheimer's or vascular dementia.

Cognitive symptoms

These are the symptoms that most people associate with dementia. Patients will frequently come to me in surgery saying that they think they are losing their mind or their "marbles" or have "completely lost the plot". Whatever words they choose, something has very definitely been lost and they are not sure why or where it's gone.

Alternatively, they may come with a relative who's concerned about forgetfulness, frequent phone calls to ask the same question, or a newfound ability to lose everything they own.

Some of the most common cognitive symptoms are:

- poor memory for names and places

- getting lost and wandering

- losing things or storing them in odd places (for example, putting their slippers in the fridge)

- loss of judgment, such as absence of awareness of danger or dressing inappropriately for the weather (an overcoat on a summer's day or lack of a raincoat during a downpour)

- declining ability to read and write and to hold a normal conversation.

Emotional symptoms

There are also losses associated with the emotional changes that can happen in dementia, with people often losing the ability to respond appropriately in social situations and in public. This is usually because of a combination of the following common emotional symptoms:

- becoming easily agitated about small things and making mountains out of molehills

- paranoid ideas about people that lead to suspicion and sometimes accusing behaviour

- sexually disinhibited talk or overfamiliarity with people

- impatience with people or with the social convention of waiting in line

- aggression

- inappropriate laughter or tears.

These symptoms can put a real strain on relationships, as it's hard not to take harsh comments or public humiliation personally.

Functional symptoms

We used to go to my grandmother's for Sunday lunch every week, and despite the odd swig of sherry while she prepared it, she still made a mean roast beef and legendary Yorkshire puddings. As her dementia developed – and I only realized this later with the luxury of hindsight – her ability to coordinate the timing of the meat and different types of vegetable started to abandon her. We'd arrive to find my grandpa hastily peeling forgotten spuds. Eventually, something that she'd prided herself on lovingly providing for her family for years was beyond her. Normally capable people gradually losing the ability to perform tasks they've done all their adult lives is the third type of loss that can signal the onset of dementia. And it can affect everything from cooking to washing and dressing, housework, gardening, and, most dangerously for others, driving.

Ten warning signs for dementia

- Memory loss that starts to affect the way you are able to live life.
- Problems with planning things or in problem solving.
- Inability to complete normally familiar tasks.
- Becoming disorientated about time and place.
- Trouble with words when speaking or writing.
- Always losing things and not being able to retrace your steps.
- Poor judgment, especially when it comes to money.
- Social withdrawal.
- Mood changes.
- Personality changes.

Disease-specific symptoms

Most of the symptoms we've looked at apply to all types of dementia, and there's a lot of overlap between Alzheimer's disease and vascular dementia in particular. However, there are some specific symptoms that suggest either Lewy body disease or frontotemporal dementia which are worth being aware of.

Lewy body disease

This disease shares a number of features with Parkinson's disease and so will often have symptoms that affect a person's movement. It can also cause weird thoughts and hallucinations, which can be quite distressing. The main distinguishing symptoms to look out for are:

- muscle stiffness

- slower movement

- tremors and shakiness of arms and legs

- loss of facial expression

- visual hallucinations (seeing animals or people that aren't there)

- delusions (holding strong beliefs that aren't true).

Frontotemporal dementia

Because the frontal lobes of the brain are involved with social and emotional responses and behaviour, these can be affected in this type of dementia. This will often affect a person's ability to show empathy to someone else, resulting in inappropriate comments and behaviour. Symptoms may therefore include:

- strange or sexually disinhibited behaviour

- aggression

- responses to people that seem cold and uncaring

- disinterest in personal hygiene

- repetitive or compulsive behaviour.

What next?

If you notice any of these symptoms in others or in yourself, then the next step is to check out whether or not they could be caused by dementia. In Chapter 3 we look at how to find out.

In Chapter 3 we look at how to find out.

Mythbuster

Dementia is the same as Alzheimer's disease.
As we've seen, dementia is a condition caused by a number of diseases, with Alzheimer's being just one of them.

Mild cognitive impairment (MCI)

This condition is like an intermediate stage between the normally ageing brain and full-on dementia. It affects memory and thought processes in the same way that dementia does, but it doesn't interfere with someone's ability to carry out normal daily activities. It can, however, be a sign that full-on dementia is developing, and it's reckoned that as many as 50 per cent of people with mild cognitive impairment will eventually be diagnosed with dementia, especially of the Alzheimer's type.

The normally ageing brain

It has long been known that as we get older our brain power isn't all that it used to be, with memory being one of the main faculties to deteriorate. It was thought that this was because of a loss of brain cells during the ageing process.

But scientists have now discovered that, unless we have a disease that specifically kills off our neurones, we die with about the same number of brain cells that we had when we were born. And although, between the ages of 20 and 90, our brains do lose about 10 per cent of their weight and shrink a little, this is not the reason for our cognitive decline either.

The problem, it seems, is that the cells we have stop communicating so well with each other. They have fewer connections, or synapses, to help pass messages from one neurone to the next and this seems to slow us down.

The abnormally ageing brain

So, when we move on to look at mild cognitive impairment, we find a worsening of the normal situation just mentioned. Half of the people with this condition remain stable for the rest of their lives, or even return to the normal picture above. The rest, however, go on to develop dementia within five years.

A scale has been developed that shows the various degrees of impairment that people can have on the spectrum of normal to disabling dementia. This scale, called the Global Deterioration Score for ageing and dementia (GDS), has four stages:

- Stage 1: No problems are identified by either doctors or the patient.

- Stage 2: The patient personally thinks they have a problem because, for example, they have trouble remembering names, but they perform normally on diagnostic tests.

- Stage 3: There are subtle problems with executive functions which are affecting work and social activities.

- Stage 4: The patient has obvious problems with mental processes which affect normal day-to-day tasks, such as planning and preparing meals and dealing with financial matters.

People at stage 3 are felt to fit the criteria of mild cognitive impairment, with those in stages 1 and 2 being classified as normal and stage 4 suggesting dementia.

Causes of mild cognitive impairment

No one is 100 per cent sure what causes MCI, as there is likely to be a combination of triggers for this condition rather than just one. Many of the most commonly fancied triggers are also those of dementia itself. These include furring of the arteries, excess shrinkage of brain tissue (particularly in the hippocampus where memories are formed), and protein plaque and tangle formation inside the nerve cells.

The risk factors for developing MCI again mirror those for dementia, with high blood pressure, diabetes, smoking, and lack of exercise being familiar suspects. It's also thought that lack of social and intellectual stimulation may be a factor. Where your mind is concerned, it seems to be a real case of use it or lose it.

3

First steps to finding a diagnosis

So, what do you do if you are worried that you or someone you know has dementia because they are exhibiting some or all of the symptoms we've mentioned in Chapter 2?

Whatever these symptoms are, the first port of call should be your family doctor or the family doctor of the person you are worried about. They are perfectly placed to get the ball rolling when it comes to investigating changes in mind and behaviour. One of the great privileges of being a family doctor is that you get to know someone over a long period of time. Most people do not change doctors unless they move house, so will have been known by the practice, if not the same doctor, for many years. This means that through the medical record, or, more often, the personal relationship of the doctor with their patient, the degree and significance of any changes in a person's mood, memory, or behaviour can easily be identified.

For that reason, if you are taking a friend or relative to be checked over, then it is always best to ask if they can see their usual doctor, even if that means waiting a day or so, as the process will be smoother for doctor and patient alike.

The same goes for worries at the weekend. If you live away and have some concerns about a relative's mental state, having not visited for some time, please don't panic and call the out-of-hours service unless the person is at imminent risk of harm. First, the situation may already be known to their own doctor and be in the process of being dealt with. Second, the deputizing doctor is unlikely to have any notes about the person, which will make the situation more confusing all round and may lead to snap decisions, such as a precautionary but inappropriate hospital admission.

Likewise, if the person has come to stay with you, taking them to see your own doctor as a temporary resident will not be helpful either, unless, again, you consider the situation is a true emergency.

So, continuity of care is paramount in dementia.

At that first appointment it would be helpful to bring along some notes detailing your concerns. Often, once people have sat down in the consulting room they forget half of what they wanted to say, which may be the critical half that gives the doctor the diagnosis, or at least the clues to planning further investigations. Taking along notes from others who have concerns about you but can't be there can also be helpful as it gives a more objective view on things.

For some people, it can be very embarrassing to go to the doctor about memory problems, and they will often deny what the person who's brought them says and play down their symptoms.

But honesty is vital in this situation. If the doctor has all the facts, they can work out what is and isn't going on far more quickly. That could be to reassure you that you are right, that this isn't dementia after all, but perhaps just part of normal ageing or, at worst, mild cognitive impairment. Or if they feel there is a possibility that the symptoms suggest dementia, then they can arrange further tests as soon as possible and start treatment, perhaps before it's too late to have an effect.

So, whether it's about you or someone else, be honest and give the doctor all and any information you think is relevant.

Your appointment at the doctor's

The medical history

At medical school it was drummed into us that 80 per cent of a diagnosis can be made from taking a good medical history. A thorough physical examination will then pretty much complete the picture, with blood tests, checks of various bodily fluids, and x-ray images of the patient's insides putting the icing on the diagnostic cake.

So when you go for your appointment, be prepared to answer a lot of questions, as we have a set list of things that we will be keen to cover. And given that most consultations are only ten minutes long, don't be surprised if you're asked to come back another day to be grilled some more if necessary.

Initially, the focus will be on the presenting complaint, with the doctor asking a nice open question such as, "What can I do for you today?" This is your chance to get it all off your chest and discuss whatever it is that is worrying you about yourself or someone else.

Next come questions to tease out a bit more detail about how things have unfolded. These questions will be aimed at finding out:

- what the concerning symptoms are

- how long symptoms have been going on for

- if the symptoms have changed since they started

- what effects symptoms are having (specifically on ability to cook, clean the house, do the shopping, wash and bathe, manage money, and drive a car)

- a possible obvious cause (such as a recent head injury, an infection, or depression).

The doctor will also enquire about other vital background information such as:

- family history of memory disorders or dementia

- details of prescribed and over-the-counter medications (as some side effects can mimic dementia by causing confusion)

- usual levels of alcohol consumption and whether you partake of the odd cigarette or two.

The physical check-up
Next comes the physical examination, although this may happen at a subsequent appointment if the medical history has been very detailed or complicated and everyone is worn out by the experience.

The examination will involve a quick all-over check-up but will focus on circulation, the nervous system, and signs of alcohol overuse. So be prepared to have:

- your blood pressure and pulse checked

- your heart and lungs listened to with a stethoscope

- your belly prodded

- your muscle power, skin sensitivity, and reflexes checked to assess your nervous system.

Alongside these hands-on physical tests, the doctor will also have been carrying out a psychological examination by simply taking note of the way in which questions have been answered and whether the story has changed at all and by looking for signs of irritability, low mood, or any inappropriate or disinhibited behaviour.

Other tests
Once these simple checks have been completed in the surgery, a series of blood and other tests may be ordered. These will be used to help rule in or out the various physical causes of dementia and confusion.

Blood tests will be checking for:

- signs of infection

- anaemia

- liver or kidney disease

- diabetes

- thyroid gland upset

- levels of blood minerals (such as sodium, potassium, and calcium)

- levels of vitamins (particularly vitamin B12 and folate).

If an infection is suspected, then a urine sample or chest x-ray may be asked for, and, depending on the findings of enquiry and examination of the circulatory system, an ECG (heart tracing) may also be on the list of required investigations.

Once all of this has been done, you will probably have a week or so's breather while the results are collated, before having a review appointment back at the surgery. If the tests give a possible explanation for your symptoms, then treatment will begin at that next appointment. So, for example, if you have bacteria in your urine, antibiotics will be prescribed, or if there are signs of infection on your x-ray, you'll get a dose of something for that too.

If there's a deficiency in iron or vitamins, or if there's a thyroid gland abnormality, then further investigations of this may be needed. And if your blood sugar shows evidence of diabetes, then sorting that out will be the priority.

If, however, all the tests are normal, the next stage of investigation will feature tests of memory and brain function and a likely scan of your brain as well. And the first port of call for these will again be your doctor's surgery.

Cognitive tests
There are several tests available and different doctors will have their favourites. They are all designed to work out

which exact areas of a person's memory and thought processes are affected.

Each test will involve different types of question which will probe the various mental capacities under scrutiny. A lot of people find these tests very embarrassing to complete in front of a doctor they may have known for years, or a relative or friend they don't want to look daft in front of or hear say, "There, Mum, you do have problems – told you so!"

It's assumed that we all know what day it is, who the prime minister is, and which building we are sitting in, and people can feel extremely ashamed if they don't know the answers to such seemingly simple questions.

When I carry out these assessments in surgery, I always try to put the person at ease by saying that there are some really silly tasks and questions coming up and not to be worried about getting some of them wrong as most other people make lots of mistakes too.

Categories of question

- *Orientation to time and place* – what year is it? Which city do you live in?
- *Short-term memory* – listen to this address and repeat it back. I will ask you it again later.
- *Attention span and calculation* – count backwards subtracting three each time or spell "world" backwards.
- *Recall* – what was the address I told you earlier?
- *Language* – name two objects on the doctor's desk.
- *Repetition* – repeat a phrase word for word.

- *Complex commands* – carry out a short task such as picking up something, moving it, and placing it somewhere else.
- *Visuo-spatial functioning* – copy a pattern or draw an object.

The tests only take five to ten minutes to complete and will give an idea of areas of a person's brain functioning that need further investigation. Each test gives a score out of a possible total that someone could achieve if they had no cognitive difficulties, so the severity of a person's symptoms can be judged by how low a score they achieve.

Brain imaging

The final part of the diagnostic jigsaw is a referral to the x-ray department for a scan of your brain. There are two types of scan that are commonly used.

CT scans

CT is the abbreviation for computerized tomography, which involves lying down on a table while the scanner, a short tunnel that looks like an enormous doughnut, moves over your head to take images of your brain structure. These images are taken in slices so that the different bits of brain anatomy at various levels can be looked at in great detail.

A CT scanner uses x-rays which pass through your body's tissues to different degrees depending on how dense that tissue is. So, for example, they pass through soft tissues such as the brain more easily than through harder structures such as bone, but not as easily as they do through your blood or the air spaces in your lungs. This allows the x-ray specialist (radiologist) to be able to identify the different parts of the brain structure and any changes to it caused by disease processes. They know what a normal brain looks like, so the images generated can be analysed for change.

Occasionally, they might inject a dye into a vein in your arm while you're having the scan done. This will make some of the structures they are looking at glow brighter in the final images and give a clearer picture of what's going on.

It's a quick and painless investigation (unless you have the injection, and even that's not too bad) which is over in about twenty minutes. For those who are extremely claustrophobic, or too agitated to lie still, sedation with medication is possible but avoided unless absolutely necessary. Although you will be alone in a room inside the scanner, the technician (radiographer) will be in contact with you via an intercom.

MRI scans
These are sometimes preferred to CT scans because they give clearer images of the blood vessels deep in the brain.

Magnetic resonance imaging (MRI) differs from CT because, instead of x-rays being used to capture the images of your brain, magnetic fields and radio waves are used. These pictures take longer to capture, so you are likely to be in the scanner for around forty-five minutes. The scanner is also very noisy, so you will be given headphones.

Once the scan is over, the images of the sections of your brain will be studied by the radiologist and a report sent to your family doctor in around one week.

Why scan the brain?

Although doctors can gain some useful diagnostic information from these types of scans – for example, shrinkage of the outer layer of the brain and signs of blood clots or poor circulation – they are mainly used to look for other possible causes of your symptoms, such as brain tumours, strokes, and excess fluid in the brain (hydrocephalus).

Putting the whole picture together

Once your doctor has all your test results, they will be able to give you a good idea about the cause of your symptoms. It may be that they've come across a treatable cause and will refer you to the relevant hospital specialist. Or it may be that the tests are conclusive for dementia.

If this is the case, then they will talk to you and your family or carers about the next step. This usually involves referral to a memory clinic, which will carry out more detailed tests to determine the type of dementia and advise about treatments. It may be, however, that you feel that having the diagnosis is enough for now, and because of other health complaints or general frailty, you may not want to be put through more cognitive tests or whizzed into more high-tech scanners.

If that's the case, your doctor will talk about the support that's available when the dementia starts to prevent you from carrying out normal daily activities (more of which later).

4

At the memory clinic

Specialist-run memory clinics have a number of different purposes:

- early identification and diagnosis of memory problems and the different types of dementia

- comprehensive, detailed investigation

- support and advice for patients, relatives, and other carers

- consideration of medication

- advice about other agencies and charities that can provide social, psychological, and practical help and support.

They are therefore well worth going to if your doctor refers you.

The clinics are staffed by a variety of different types of specialist doctor. These could be consultants in care of the elderly medicine, old-age psychiatry, or neurology (problems with the nervous system). The team will also include clinical psychologists and specialist nurses.

Further tests

They will put you through some even more rigorous cognitive tests to fine-tune the diagnosis and work out exactly what your brain is having difficulty doing. They may also arrange for you to have more detailed brain scans to confirm which of the different types of dementia you have.

These scans are usually PET scans, which stands for positron emission tomography. MRIs and CT scans take black-and-white snaps of your brain's structure, but PET scans provide multicoloured images not only of your brain's structure but also of its activity.

Positrons are radioactive particles that can be attached to a chemical that's normally used by the body, called a radiotracer. In the case of studies into dementia, this chemical is a type of sugar that the brain uses for energy. This radiotracer, with its piggy-backing positrons, is injected into your veins, swallowed as a pill, or inhaled as a vapour before you go into the scanner.

Once the radiotracer arrives in your brain, the positrons give off energy called gamma rays, which are then picked up by the scanner and turned into multicoloured images. Areas of greatest brain activity are reddest and brightest in colour and are called hotspots, whereas those areas where the brain is not really doing much look bluer and colder.

PET scans take a long time to perform because you have to wait for the radiotracer to navigate your system and arrive in your brain before the scan can even begin. The radiotracer's journey takes about an hour and then the scan itself can take a similar amount of time.

It's worth the inconvenience, though. These scans are an excellent way to allow doctors to differentiate between Alzheimer's disease and frontotemporal dementia because of the different patterns these conditions generate when looked at in the scanner. This allows your specialist to reach a specific diagnosis quickly and tailor treatment accordingly.

Other services

Memory clinics not only help to arrive at a diagnosis quickly and start appropriate medication, but they are also a hub for signposting people to other types of ongoing care. We will look at what sorts of help are available in Chapter 7.

5

Medical treatments

In our high-tech twenty-first-century world, it's very easy to assume that medical science will be able to come up with some sort of cure for all the diseases that nature throws at us. A century ago even simple infections were major killers, but now we have antibiotics that will fend them off within a week. And with heart bypass surgery commonplace, Olympic-standard artificial limbs available, and even face transplants now possible, it is hard to believe that there are still some conditions that we cannot cure. Sadly, there is still not a pill for every ill and there are some people we just can't make better.

And unfortunately dementia – for now anyway – is one of those incurable conditions. But there are a number of things doctors have up their sleeves that can help to improve its symptoms and some exciting research developments that may offer real hope for the future.

Pills

There are four different drugs on the market that can be prescribed to treat the symptoms of dementia. So far only specialists in memory clinics have been able to start these treatments, but it is likely that family doctors will soon be able to start them too.

These medicines have been specifically developed to help the symptoms of Alzheimer's disease, but many specialists will also try them when people have mixed dementia. Again, none of these medicines is a cure for the condition, but they can all help to minimize its effects for a while and improve the quality of life of someone with dementia.

Like most prescription medicines, they all have unpronounceable, whacky names that are difficult to get your tongue around. The four currently on the market are donepezil, galantamine, rivastigmine, and memantine.

How do they work?

The first three drugs on the list – donepezil, galantamine, and rivastigmine – are what are called anticholinesterase inhibitors. They work on one of the chemical transmitters in the brain, called acetylcholine.

Acetylcholine passes messages between nerve cells in areas of the brain that are involved in memory; in Alzheimer's disease, there is less of this chemical around and memory is consequently affected.

Anticholinesterase inhibitors prevent what acetylcholine there is from being broken down. This raises the level of this transmitter and symptoms can improve.

Memantine works on a different chemical transmitter, called glutamate. When brain cells become damaged by

 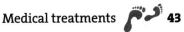

dementia, glutamate leaks out of them and disrupts the processes of memory and learning that are being carried out by other cells. By blocking the receptors for glutamate on these other cells, this interference can be stopped and the cells can do their job as normal. This helps people with Alzheimer's to be able to think more clearly.

How long does treatment carry on for?

It's reckoned that these medicines help around 50 to 60 per cent of the people who are given them, with the benefits lasting around six months. This can mean that at best their symptoms improve or at the very least their symptoms are stabilized and don't get any worse while they are on the treatment.

Researchers have also had promising results from studies looking at long-term treatment with these medicines. They've found that if people stay on them for up to a year, it can slow down the rate at which memory symptoms get worse and also lead to improvements in the way people are able to carry out everyday activities such as washing, dressing, and cooking.

Unfortunately, if the drugs don't help at all after a trial of a few months, then they are unlikely ever to and will be stopped.

The table opposite lists each of the drugs alongside the ways in which they can be taken and possible early side effects. For the majority of people, any side effects are minimal and don't last for more than a week or two.

Name of drug	Method of taking	Possible side effects
Donepezil (Aricept)	Ordinary tablets Melt-in-the-mouth tablets	Sickness, diarrhoea, headaches, dizziness, weird dreams and hallucinations, poor sleep, tiredness, agitation
Galantamine (Reminyl and Galsya)	Ordinary tablets Liquid Slow-release tablets	Sickness, diarrhoea, indigestion, loss of appetite, weight loss, high blood pressure, slowing of pulse, headache, dizziness, hallucinations
Rivastigmine (Exelon)	Capsules Liquid Patches	Sickness, diarrhoea, indigestion, loss of appetite, weight loss, slow pulse, dizziness, headache, drowsiness, agitation, anxiety, tremor, confusion, insomnia, symptoms of Parkinson's disease
Memantine (Ebixa)	Tablets Liquid	Constipation, high blood pressure, shortness of breath, headache, dizziness, drowsiness

What about the other types of dementia?

At the moment, drugs for Alzheimer's disease are the only specific treatments available. They can help with mixed dementia, as already mentioned, and although they are not licensed for use in Lewy body disease, they can improve the symptoms of challenging behaviour that can happen in this condition.

Vascular dementia can be slowed down by treating the underlying causes, such as raised blood pressure, diabetes, and high cholesterol levels, and by stopping smoking.

Treatment of distressing symptoms

Despite the lack of specific treatment options, doctors are able to prescribe other drugs to help when someone with dementia becomes depressed, their behaviour becomes extremely difficult, or they seem to be in constant distress.

However, before prescribing anything, an assessment should be made of who the symptoms are most distressing to: the person with dementia or their carers. It is not appropriate to prescribe potentially harmful medicines to someone simply to give their carers a quieter time. In fact, it's been found that prescribing antipsychotic drugs to control the behaviour of people with dementia results directly in almost 2,000 unnecessary deaths per year.

These medicines should only be used as a last resort and only when all possible alternative strategies have been tried and an underlying cause such as pain has been excluded. These strategies will be considered in Chapter 6.

Mythbuster

Once you're diagnosed with dementia your life is over. Although there is no cure for dementia and people are affected by it in different ways, there are plenty of medical, psychological, and social treatments that can help people maintain a good and meaningful quality of life, potentially for many years.

6

Natural and alternative remedies

Tap the words "natural remedies for memory loss" into any internet search engine and you'll be greeted with page after page of holistic offerings from Mother Nature's medicine chest. And her chest must be more than ample as it seems to be bursting with cures for poor memory, lack of concentration, and full-on dementia, all gathered from organic sources and passed on with the seemingly magical wisdom of our ancient forebears.

The trouble is that for many of the treatments there does seem to be far more magic than medicine on offer. Some of the lists of medicinal plant life read more like ingredients for a potion Harry Potter might wizard up to paralyse a marauding troll than serious attempts to improve cognitive function. And on one site the curative list of rosemary, sage, walnuts, almonds, and apples would be more at home in a Jamie Oliver recipe for a deliciously crunchy autumn salad than a medical textbook.

So, is the idea of treating dementia more naturally just a load of hocus-pocus? Or is there some truth in what those touting complementary therapies have to say? And can any of them do more harm than good? Well, unless you have an allergy to nuts, the chances of an almond giving you side effects is pretty non-existent. But it is a sensible question and many of us wrongly assume that because something is organic and natural it doesn't carry the same risks as prescription medicines.

Fortunately, some studies have looked at the effectiveness of these treatments and the possible downsides of each, allowing sensible decisions to be made. So here's a review of five complementary therapies that seem to be mentioned particularly frequently on the internet.

Ginkgo biloba
This plant extract tops the charts for most lauded complementary remedy for dementia.

Where does it come from?
Ginkgo or maidenhair trees date back to the prehistoric forests grazed by the dinosaurs. They grow all over the world but were particularly popular in temple gardens in the Far East. They can reach a height of a whopping 40 metres and live for thousands of years, the oldest on record having survived three and a half millennia.

What's in it?
Ginkgo leaves contain two chemicals called flavonoids and terpenoids, which are believed to be antioxidants. (Antioxidants mop up potentially dangerous free radical

molecules believed to cause cell damage and lead to cancer and ageing.)

How does it work?
As well as preventing cell damage, extract from the leaves is also believed to increase blood flow to the brain.

Any side effects or drug interactions?
There are no significant side effects, but it can potentially interact with a number of prescription medications such as antidepressants, drugs for epilepsy and high blood pressure, and those used to thin the blood (anticoagulants and aspirin).

What's the verdict?
Long believed to be able to enhance memory and reverse some of the symptoms of dementia, a large-scale piece of research in 2010, which analysed combined results from a number of studies, finally confirmed its effectiveness scientifically.

Vitamin E

Where does it come from?
It is found naturally in a number of oils such as sunflower oil, in almonds and hazelnuts, and in fruit and vegetables, including pumpkins, turnips, tomatoes, avocados, asparagus, sweet potatoes, mangoes, and kiwi fruit.

What's in it?
Again, like gingko, it contains antioxidants.

 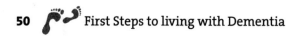

How does it work?

It is thought that its antioxidant action slows down the progression of nerve cell damage in dementia.

Any side effects or drug interactions?

Some people develop sickness, diarrhoea, and muscle weakness. Vitamin E can interact with anticoagulant drugs such as warfarin and clopidogrel to cause bruising and prolonged bleeding.

What's the verdict?

The suggestion that vitamin E could help in Alzheimer's mostly came from animal studies. When scientists look at results in real people, there is no evidence that it makes a difference.

Huperzine A

Where does it come from?

This catchily named plant extract comes from a type of moss called *Huperzia serrata* and has been a staple of Chinese medicine for centuries.

What's in it?

The chemical huperzine A has a similar anticholinesterase action to drugs such as donepezil and rivastigmine.

How does it work?

It works in the same way as the prescribed medicines by increasing the natural levels of acetylcholine in a sufferer's brain.

Any side effects or interactions?
It can cause stomach upset, chest and throat tightness, a slower heart rate, and insomnia. It cannot be used at the same time as prescribed anticholinesterase inhibitors or treatments for the eye disease glaucoma.

What's the verdict?
Some researchers have achieved very promising results with this supplement, showing that it can improve memory and reduce disability from dementia. However, at the moment there's not enough evidence to convince people to recommend it as a first-line treatment.

VITACOG
A combination of B vitamins, including B6, B12, and folic acid.

Where does it come from?
This combination was part of a scientific study carried out at Oxford University using supplements of these vitamins. They occur naturally in a wide variety of food sources, including meat, yeast extracts such as Marmite, green vegetables such as asparagus, broccoli, and spinach, dairy products, fish, and cereals.

What's in it?
The vitamins themselves are the active ingredients. Having low levels of these vitamins is known to increase the risk of Alzheimer's disease and vascular dementia. High levels of these vitamins are believed to slow the rate of both brain shrinkage and memory decline.

How does it work?
These vitamins lower the level of a protein called homocysteine, which not only damages the small blood vessels around the brain but is also toxic to nerve cells themselves.

Any side effects or interactions?
Side effects are minimal other than the usual tummy upsets that popping almost any pill can cause. There are potential interactions with iron tablets and anticoagulants.

What's the verdict?
A fair amount of success has been found with this combination of vitamins, with some researchers showing a 30 per cent reduction in homocysteine levels and a corresponding halt in cognitive decline.

Medical foods
Since 2010 the newspapers have carried a number of stories about miracle milkshakes for curing Alzheimer's. Two that have had particular mention and are currently under development by different companies are Souvenaid and Axona.

What's in them?
Souvenaid contains a variety of ingredients but especially omega-3 fatty acids, uridine, choline, and B vitamins.

Axona is made of caprylic triglyceride, which is derived from coconut oil and has been used in the cosmetics industry.

How do they work?

Souvenaid's mix of ingredients helps nerve cells to form new connections (synapses) to replace those that are lost in Alzheimer's disease.

Axona works by providing the brain of someone with Alzheimer's disease an alternative source of energy to glucose (which our brains all normally metabolize). This helps because in Alzheimer's the brain stops being able to use glucose so well and therefore starts to run out of steam.

Any side effects or interactions?

Studies so far have not uncovered any significant side effects or interactions with either of these foods, although it is recommended that Axona is used with caution in people with diabetes.

What's the verdict?

Both are still being evaluated experimentally, but results are promising and it is likely that they will both prove effective in helping people with mild to moderate dementia.

Other complementary therapies

Reminiscence therapy

When my grandmother began to develop dementia, one of the things that became most obvious was that although she didn't have a clue where she'd just put her slippers, or even what our names were, she could tell us about her experiences as a wartime nursing auxiliary as if she'd finished her last shift that morning.

Reminiscence therapy is based on the fact that most people with dementia are like my grandmother and have vivid memories from the past that can be tapped into to improve mood, well-being, and relationships with their families, carers, and the other professionals helping to look after them.

Therapy can be carried out one-to-one or as part of a group and will involve the use of photographs, cine films and videos, scrapbooks, and music – in fact, anything that may jog a memory and develop a discussion about a familiar topic. In one project, reminiscences were used to design a room in a care home to make it look familiar.

Although this is a great way to improve patient-centred care, it must be remembered that not all reminiscences are happy ones, and bad memories have to be dealt with sensitively and not just brushed under the carpet. It's also important to respect the person's wishes if they say they don't want to try this type of activity.

Suggestions for reminiscence activities

Music
Play tapes and CDs of favourite pieces of music or those with specific relevance, such as music that was danced to, played at the person's wedding, or popular at the time of a first date. Then talk about it and any associated memories about people or places that it evokes.

Visual
Photographs from family albums, or books of old pictures of the town where the person lived or grew up

can be useful here. Old movies or newsreels can also be a good way to start reminiscences of a period of their lives that a person most remembers.

Smell and taste
Use favourite foods or drinks to stimulate discussion about visits to special places, events, or the people they used to share them with.

Touch
Items of clothing and ornaments from the past can also be used, along with treasured jewellery or a loved one's medals.

These prompts can be used by carers to get to know someone or by friends and relatives to start a chat about parts of the person's life they still remember.

Reality orientation

This type of therapy has been shown to help reduce confusion and help stop troubling behaviours in people with dementia. It can be particularly beneficial in care homes and hospitals but can also be used at home if you have someone with dementia living with you.

The aim is to orientate the person to current place and time, and to the names, identities, and caring roles of the people around them. In short, it tries to enable people to know where and who they and those around them are, so as to reduce uncertainty and anxiety.

Examples would include:

- having a board on display with the day, date, next meal, and weather written on it

- mounting large calendar clocks on the wall

- buying daily, up-to-date newspapers

- displaying the names of rooms on doors, with the person's own name labelling their bedroom.

Critics of reality orientation worry that being corrected about situations can actually make people feel worse. For example, telling someone they can't go home to their husband because he died ten years ago can be very distressing for someone who has forgotten about his death and may therefore react to the news as they would the first time they heard it.

Specal therapy
So, in contrast, other therapies such as SPECAL (Specialized Early Care for Alzheimer's) have been developed. With this approach, there are three golden rules:

- Don't ask questions.

- Listen to the expert – the person with dementia – and learn from them.

- Don't contradict.

 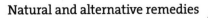

The aim of these rules is to avoid the person becoming distressed by being challenged by questions their memory won't help them answer and to listen to the questions they themselves are asking and try to answer them from their point of view and not our own.

Psychologist Oliver James, writing in *The Guardian* newspaper in 2008, used this example taken from the experiences of Penny Garner, developer of the SPECAL approach, to highlight its benefits both for carers and the people they are looking after:

> *Garner's ideas evolved as a result of caring for her mother, Dorothy Johnson, when she developed Alzheimer's. One day, they were sitting together in a doctor's waiting room when out of the blue Dorothy said, "Has our flight been called yet?" Garner was mystified and played for time. Her mother anxiously looked around and said, "We don't want to miss it, where's our hand luggage?"*
>
> *Suddenly, Garner realised what was happening. Her mother had always loved air travel and Dorothy was making sense of this crowded waiting situation by assuming they were in a departure lounge. When Garner responded with "All our luggage has been checked in, we've just got our handbags," her mother visibly relaxed.*

Despite the obvious benefits of this approach in its ability to reduce anxiety in someone with dementia and avoid confrontation with the carer, critics have voiced concerns that this method disempowers people with dementia because, by not being told the truth about situations they are in, they are prevented from being involved in any proper decision making.

Having watched my mum struggling to correct my grandmother when she repeatedly mistook me for her own son (my uncle) when he was a boy, I can see some merit in avoiding confrontation. But although we may need to choose our battles and not argue about everything, it cannot be good to deceive people about reality, as this could instead add to confusion.

To use the example given by Oliver James above, if someone comes to see me in surgery because they have a bad cough, and their carer has colluded with them that they are at the airport waiting for their departure gate to open, how will they respond when the person they see, who must surely be an airline steward, asks them to take their clothes off so he can examine their chest, rather than giving them the peanuts and in-flight gin and tonic they were expecting?

Aromatherapy

Now to a treatment that's far less contentious. The use of aromatic plant oils to promote well-being has been around since biblical times and there is loads of evidence for their benefits to health.

In dementia, these oils, which can be either breathed in or applied to the skin, can help with agitation, restlessness, antisocial behaviour, confusion, and insomnia. It's not really known how these treatments work, as many patients with dementia have lost their sense of smell, but they are a safe (when used by trained practitioners) and undoubtedly effective way of helping people who have some of dementia's more difficult symptoms.

Aromatic oils shown to help in dementia

- Lavender
- Basil
- Chamomile
- Coriander
- Lemon
- Lemon balm
- Neroli

Bright light therapy

Sleep patterns can be really messed up for people with dementia, with "sundowning" being a particular problem (see Chapter 7). Traditionally prescribed drug treatments are potentially harmful, so this treatment is an option if simple bedtime routines don't help.

It involves using a lightbox that's around thirty times brighter than an ordinary bulb, with the person sitting in front of it for between thirty minutes and two hours per day. Using this treatment daily can help people with dementia to develop better sleep patterns and it has also been shown to promote better-quality sleep and to help lift low mood.

Music therapy

This therapy uses musical tunes, rhythms, instruments, and singing to improve a person's sense of well-being. Music has a great power to affect our thoughts and feelings. Which of us hasn't at some point leapt up during a rock song to strum away on air guitar or croon along into a hairbrush microphone? And it's rare that a piece of music won't have reduced us to tears at some time in our lives.

In dementia, receptivity to music can continue long after other mental processes such as concentration and memory have been lost, so the power of music to evoke these feelings can be used to communicate with people even when they struggle to make sense of things at all other times.

Music therapy

In his book *Musicophilia*, neurologist Oliver Sacks tells the lovely story of eighty-year-old Bessie T. She was a former blues singer but now struggled with Alzheimer's disease, which had left her with such severe amnesia that she couldn't hold anything in her mind for more than a minute. When there was a talent show in the hospital where she lived, she and her music therapist practised some songs together and, on the day, she performed beautifully and with great feeling, remembering all of the words. Yet just a few moments later, after she had stepped away from the microphone, she couldn't recall having sung at all.

7

Dealing with troublesome symptoms

As dementia progresses, a number of types of behaviour may develop that can be really stressful for carers. These behaviours take a variety of forms, but there are definite patterns that we see in many people with dementia. Most are mild and can be dealt with without professional help, but they can become extreme and need input from the person's doctor or specialist community nurse.

These problems generally fit into the symptom categories that we've seen already: cognitive, emotional, and functional. But it should also be remembered that some symptoms aren't a direct result of the dementia itself but are due to pain or distress from some other cause (such as the symptoms of arthritis) and the dementia has taken away the ability to communicate this more straightforwardly.

 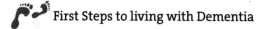

Cognitive

Wandering

Wandering can be the most problematic behaviour in this category as it can put the person at risk not only of getting lost but also of injury from other hazards such as traffic and, if it happens at night, muggers. I've had patients who have been troubled by both, including a woman who was picked up by the police wandering in her nightie and slippers along the central reservation of a nearby motorway.

But this high-risk behaviour is not simply designed to worry carers or keep the police from twiddling their thumbs. It's most often caused by a variety of genuine factors:

- Memory lapses – midway through one task, the person forgets what they were up to and thinks they should be somewhere else. Or it may be that they are going back to the past and head off, convinced they need to be at work, but get lost on the way.

- Their environment may simply be too busy or noisy, or just not where they want to be, so they wander off to escape.

- Excess energy and boredom – just because someone has dementia doesn't mean they don't need exercise!

Suggestions to help prevent wandering:

- Keep the person stimulated and active, and go out for regular walks with them to cause natural tiredness.

- If it's their own house, try obscuring the front door by hanging a curtain in front it, so it's not so obviously an exit.

- Inform helpful neighbours and local shopkeepers that the person is prone to wandering.

- Sew name tags into clothes and nightwear, so the person can be identified when found.

- Ask their family doctor to check that there's no physical problem or drug reaction responsible.

Repetitive behaviour

This is another common behaviour that can get right under your skin if you are a carer. It might take the form of having questions endlessly repeated to you, continuously rearranging the objects in a room, or seemingly endless phone calls.

Again, memory can play a part in causing repetitive behaviour – the person simply forgets they've already asked you something. But it can be because they are in distress and trying to communicate it to you in the wrong way, or simply because of boredom.

It can be helped in a number of ways:

- Go over things more slowly and deliberately and perhaps use visual aids to explain an answer.

- Ask if there's something else that's disturbing them.

- Take time out of a situation for you to cool down if things get heated, as your agitation could well be unsettling and make the repetitive behaviour worse.

 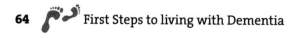

- Use an answerphone to screen calls.

- Get the doctor to check for a medical cause if the behaviour is new or worsening.

Sundowning

This problem can be exhausting for carers because it involves sleepless nights all round. Sufferers develop increasing confusion and sleeplessness each evening and end up awake and disorientated all night. They then happily nod off in the day to get some rest while the carer has to get on with normal activities before the whole process repeats itself again at sunset.

Potential remedies include:

- bright light therapy (see Chapter 6)

- avoiding caffeinated drinks such as tea and coffee after supper

- cutting down on mentally stimulating activities in the evening

- the usual medical check-up for treatable causes.

Emotional

Here, anger and irritability top the list of common symptoms. They can manifest as shouting and screaming, physically lashing out at people, and unusually rude speech.

Although disinhibition resulting from dementia may make these behaviours both more likely and perhaps more extreme, it's worth remembering that someone with dementia is as likely to be made angry by the things that annoy them as the rest of us are. And they have every right to be. As they become less able to look after themselves, it's inevitable that people will have to do more for them, but when this is done without consideration for their preferred way of doing things or without any effort to protect dignity, it's going to cause upset.

If someone stripped me off in a cold bathroom, shoved me in a shower, and poked me with a sponge on a stick, we would quickly fall out!

But there can be other underlying causes which can be helped by:

- doing unto others as we would have them do unto us (in other words, ask how they like things done and do it with concern for their comfort and personal dignity)

- asking a professional to check that the problem is not being caused by illness, depression, or pain

- maintaining a calm approach, especially when in public, to avoid things escalating.

ABC analysis

One way of trying to get to the bottom of this sort of behaviour, so that it can be minimized in future, is called the ABC analysis of behaviour, where:

- A involves observing the situations that *activate* the behaviour
- B stands for noting exactly what the *behaviour* involves
- C is identifying the *consequences* of that behaviour.

By working out what triggered the behaviour, how it developed, and any aggravating factors, such as

 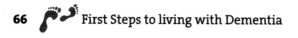

other people's unhelpful responses, strategies can be developed to help prevent or reduce its severity in future.

Functional

Incontinence
Unfortunately, people with dementia can become doubly incontinent of both bowels and waterworks, but it's urinary incontinence that's most common. The causes can be sorted into four main categories:

- problems with the bladder itself, such as bladder muscle irritability, a weak outflow muscle because of slack pelvic floor muscles after childbirth, and an enlarged prostate gland in men

- problems that affect how the bladder or kidneys work, including urinary tract infections (cystitis), diabetes, constipation, and the effects of various medications

- problems with the brain's control of the bladder, which can be a direct result of the dementia itself

- problems actually getting to the loo, because of mobility problems or forgetting where it is.

Getting around this issue involves working out the cause and addressing it. This may mean a trip to the doctor's to review pills or check for water infections and constipation, or simply either having better labelling on the bathroom door or encouraging more frequent trips to the toilet.

Falls

Although recurrent falls can be an early sign of dementia in some people, they become much more common as the condition worsens, with around 50 per cent of sufferers having at least one fall a year. That's twice the frequency of falls in the general elderly population.

Falls are caused by dementia-related damage to the brain's coordination and balance systems, the effects of various prescribed drugs (which can cause blood pressure to drop on standing up), and absentmindedly tripping over rugs and furniture that the person forgot were there.

Prevention might involve working on balance with a physiotherapist, removing hazards from the room and making an easier route from chair to door, asking the family doctor to review medications, and having ramps and rails fitted.

Mythbuster

Everyone with dementia becomes aggressive.
Angry and aggressive behaviour can be a symptom for some people with dementia, but by no means does it affect everyone. It can often be prevented by improving a person's surroundings, better communication, and ensuring they are always treated with respect.

Finding the right care

The care needs of people with dementia will be as different as the people themselves. They will depend on the degree of functional disability that the condition causes, alter as the dementia progresses, and vary according to the desire and ability of a person's family to help. But one thing is certain: with doctors having very little up their sleeves in the way of treatments, the social needs of someone with dementia will be the prime concern.

A number of other health and social care professionals may well be able to help, and charities also offer care and support for sufferers and those who look after them. The provision of these services will differ from place to place but examples would include the following.

Healthcare

- Community nurses can support people who wish to live independently but are at risk of falls or hospital admission. They can advise about access to other services and safety measures (such as pendant alarms) and also play a vital role in monitoring a person's condition by offering check-ups and giving flu jabs.

- Community pharmacists can review side effects of medicines and arrange for pills to be put into blister packs to make them simpler to take.

- Specialist memory nurses are often attached to the local memory clinic. They provide follow-up for people at home and offer advice to families, carers, and family doctors who have particular concerns about a patient.

- Physiotherapists can work with people who are at risk of falls to improve their stability so as to allow them to remain active.

- Occupational therapists can have an important role in enabling people to maintain and improve their ability to carry out everyday tasks. They can also advise about home adaptations such as stair rails and walk-in showers that can make life easier and safer for those with dementia.

Social care
This type of care might include:

- help at home with shopping, laundry, and cleaning

- home care, which may involve washing, dressing, and preparation of meals

- round-the-clock care in either sheltered housing or a care home

- meals on wheels.

Charities (see Appendix B) and your family doctor or specialist can advise about how these sources of care can be accessed.

Charities
Much of the support for sufferers and their carers is provided by charities and other voluntary organizations. This can be in the general form of lunch clubs for the elderly in the church hall or befriending schemes run from the local health centre, but it can also be very specifically provided for those affected by dementia. Examples include:

- befriending schemes

- carers' support groups

- memory cafés, where anyone concerned about difficulties with memory can drop in for advice and information

- "singing for the brain" music therapy sessions.

A list of charity websites is included in Appendix B.

Everyone with dementia needs to be in a nursing home.
Many people with dementia can safely be cared for in their own homes until the disease is extremely advanced, depending on the ability of family and friends to be involved and with input from health and social care workers.

 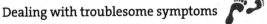

8

Legal and financial help for those with dementia

It's very important in life to feel that you have a voice that matters and that people will respect your wishes about running your own life the way you want it to be run. This applies not only to choices about lifestyle but, more importantly, to decisions about your finances, your living arrangements, and the type of healthcare treatments you receive.

That can become very difficult if you develop any of the diseases that lead to dementia, because, as we've seen, as they get worse they take away the capacity for normal reasoning, planning, and pretty much any meaningful decision-making ability at all.

There are two vital legal documents that can allow you to feel you have some control over what will and won't be done to you and with your affairs as you become more incapacitated: a living will and a lasting power of attorney.

And they can both be set up while you are still well enough to make decisions for yourself.

Living will
A living will, sometimes called an advance directive, is a statement about the medical treatments that you do and don't want if you become unable to make your own decisions in the future. They do not, as some people think, have anything to do with euthanasia.

A living will helps doctors and relatives and carers to make sensible decisions about what treatments are and aren't wanted or in your best interests if you become severely ill but cannot communicate your wishes for yourself at the time. Unfortunately, without it, things are not so straightforward and clear-cut, and I have seen a number of people put through far more invasive and gruelling treatment than was probably appropriate because their wishes weren't known in advance.

An example would be the woman with dementia who has a heart attack and whose worried carer calls the ambulance. When she then goes into cardiac arrest and there is no living will in place, the paramedics are duty-bound to start resuscitation. You do not "go gentle into that good night", as the poet Dylan Thomas put it, with an ambulance crew bouncing up and down on your ribs, pushing sharp needles into your veins, and zapping your chest with high doses of electricity through a defibrillator.

A living will is vital to prevent these situations from occurring, or to prevent potentially scary and harmful medical tests being carried out, and to allow death with dignity when it comes.

Who do you need to tell about it?

You should make sure that your family, carers, and any other medical professionals who help look after you are aware that you have completed a living will.

Once completed, it becomes a legal document, and if you have specified your refusal to be given life-saving treatment, legal action can be taken against doctors who ignore this. It is not enough, as some people have done, to have "Do not resuscitate" tattooed on your chest, as this isn't legally binding and does not provide doctors with the information they need to make a decision in an emergency situation.

Lasting power of attorney

A lasting power of attorney (LPA) allows someone you trust (the attorney) to make decisions for you when you no longer have the capacity to make them for yourself. There are two types of LPA – one for health and welfare, and the other for property and financial affairs. The health and welfare LPA allows your attorney to make decisions about where you live and the care you receive, whereas the property and financial affairs LPA allows them to look after your money matters, such as bills and benefits, and make decisions about selling your house or flat.

How to go about granting LPA

Essentially, an LPA can be made by anyone over the age of 18 who has the mental capacity to do so. In the UK the process is set up by filling in forms that are available from the Office of the Public Guardian (part of the Ministry of Justice) or online from www.direct.gov.uk. The registration process, after you've sent off the forms, costs £120 and

 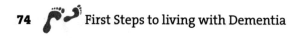

takes around nine weeks to complete. Other countries have similar arrangements, and details can be found in Appendix B.

Welfare benefits

If you have dementia or are a carer for someone who does, then you may well be eligible for financial support from the state in the form of welfare benefits. As you might expect when applying for money from the government's coffers, it's not a straightforward process and may feel like having to prise the cash from between their tightly clenched fingers.

There are a lot of forms to fill in and they will also want supporting information from doctors or social workers to fully process any application, so the procedure isn't always a quick one. But it could well be worth it and you can get advice on what you may be eligible for and help with the paperwork from Alzheimer's charities, the Citizens Advice Bureau, and various other local benefits advice agencies.

9

Can dementia be prevented?

Spend any time in a clinic with a fully paid-up member of any of the health professions and chances are that at some point they will go on about how you should be doing more exercise, swallowing less fat, stubbing out the cigarettes for good, and taking more water with your booze. We quacks have one mantra and, like a Buddhist in the lotus position, we repeat it incessantly as if we think our life, and perhaps our entrance to the next one, will depend on it.

And, in a way, that is exactly why we do it. There is more than enough convincing evidence out there that modifying our lifestyle and dietary habits will improve our health and the quality of our life now and protect us from entering our next life before our three score and ten years are up.

The evidence is not just there for the prevention of heart disease and stroke, diabetes and obesity; there's a good chance that by looking after our bodies, we might just keep our brains healthy too and reduce the risk of dementia.

The processes that lead to dementia start when people are in their forties, so this prevention should start as early as possible. In this chapter we will look at the different lifestyle adjustments that can be made to diet, level of exercise, alcohol consumption, and smoking, as well as the evidence for whether so-called "brain training" exercises really do help to protect us from dementia.

Diet

Most of the dietary advice to help prevent dementia is the same as that to prevent heart disease, because the damage to blood vessels that can be caused by fats will affect oxygen supply not only to heart muscle but also to brain tissue.

It's also known that people who are obese (with a body mass index of over 30) in middle age have a four times greater risk of developing dementia than those who are not overweight.

The best type of diet is low in fat and high in fibre, so it will ideally feature lots of fruit and vegetables (five a day), whole grains and cereals, and not too many hamburgers.

There are two main types of fat in the foods we eat: saturated and unsaturated. High levels of saturated fats increase the level of cholesterol in our blood, which is involved in damaging blood vessels, whereas unsaturated fats can help lower your cholesterol levels.

Foods containing saturated fats	Foods containing unsaturated fats
Fatty cuts of meat	Oily fish such as salmon and fresh tuna
Sausages and pies	Avocados
Cheese, butter, and lard	Unsalted nuts such as brazils and walnuts
Full-fat milk and cream	Pumpkin and sunflower seeds
Chocolates	Olive and sunflower oils
Biscuits, cakes, and pastries	

All foods in supermarkets now carry labels that indicate the levels of fat they contain using a traffic light system, where high fat content is shown in red, moderate content in yellow, and low fat content in green.

It's obviously all right to have a treat every now and again – mine's a bacon sandwich – but treats should not form the main part of your diet. In general, men should aim for having no more than 30 grams of saturated fat per day and women only 20 grams.

High fibre foods

These are plant-based foods which can lower cholesterol, prevent constipation, and help the bowel to absorb important nutrients. They also make you feel fuller at the end of a meal and so, by controlling appetite and overall food intake, they can help you to stop putting on weight.

There are two types of fibre: insoluble and soluble.

Insoluble fibre is mostly made of a plant chemical called cellulose. Good sources include:

- wholemeal and granary bread

- potatoes with their jackets left on

- wholegrain breakfast cereals

- brown rice and wholemeal pasta

- beans, peas, and lentils

- nuts.

Soluble fibre ferments in the bowel and is what gives us wind. It helps to control blood sugar and lower cholesterol. The following foods are good sources of soluble fibre:

- fruit such as apples, pears, oranges, strawberries, and bananas

- potatoes, sweet potatoes, and onions

- broccoli and carrots.

How much fibre?

If you want to eat a healthy, balanced diet, then you need to be eating around 18 grams of fibre per day. The supermarket labels give details of how much fibre is contained in each product you buy to help you hit this target.

Salt

High intake of salt can not only put up your blood pressure and increase risk of heart disease but in older people who don't exercise much it can also increase the risk of dementia. Guidelines say that adults should have no more than 6 grams of salt per day, which is about the equivalent of a teaspoon. So you really do need to keep the salt on your dinner down to a pinch.

Mythbuster

Aluminium from saucepans can cause dementia.
Because aluminium has been associated with the protein plaques and tangles seen in Alzheimer's disease it was thought that it may be a possible cause of the disease. Research has since shown this to be highly unlikely.

Smoking

Smoking is universally bad for you. It affects your heart and lungs and is linked to all manner of different cancers. It should perhaps come as no surprise, then, that it's bad for your brain too. In fact, it's so bad that it doubles your risk of developing dementia, particularly vascular dementia and Alzheimer's disease, by damaging blood vessels and nerve cells. There is also quite a lot of evidence to suggest that even passive smoking (breathing in second-hand smoke from other people's cigarettes) can increase your risk of dementia too.

The advice here is simple: stop smoking! And if you don't smoke but live with someone who does, get them to stop on your behalf.

Unfortunately, most people find it hard to give up, and for every person who makes up their mind to quit and never puts another cigarette to their lips, there are probably half a dozen more whose cravings always get the better of them.

Thankfully, if you are in that second group of people, in the UK help is at hand on the NHS. Stop smoking clinics are available through surgeries, pharmacy stores, some libraries, and even in community centres. These provide medication on prescription to stop the cravings for another cigarette. But it's the support these clinics provide that is the key to their success, with those who have a prescription and ongoing follow-up being far more successful at stopping – and staying stopped – than those who just take the script and go it alone.

The three main types of stop smoking medication are:

- Champix: a prescription-only tablet

- Zyban: a prescription-only tablet

- nicotine replacement therapy – available from pharmacies and supermarkets in a number of forms: gum, patches, microtabs (which melt in the mouth), lozenges, inhalators, or nasal spray.

All of these treatments are as effective as each other and the smoking advisors will go through the pros and cons of each with you in clinic and tailor the best treatment they can find to suit you individually.

Exercise

Getting regular exercise is an important way of helping to prevent vascular dementia and Alzheimer's disease. This isn't the "no pain, no gain" type of exercise where you sign up for marathons, and it won't necessarily involve you forking out for an expensive gym membership or having to kit yourself out from head to toe in lycra.

 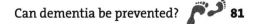

The regular exercise in question need only take the form of five half-hour brisk walks per week, with the dog or to the shops to get your milk and newspaper. In fact, as long as whatever you do puts your pulse up a little, it could include cycling, swimming, gardening, housework, or a combination of all of them. You could even try using the stairs instead of the lift when there's a choice of the two – it all adds up.

Alcohol

As we've already seen in Chapter 1, alcohol can cause its own type of dementia: Korsakoff's syndrome. It's therefore important to stick to the government's recommended guidelines of:

• 3–4 units per day for a man

• 2–3 units per day for a woman.

If you're regularly drinking more than that, then you must cut down, because not only does it mess with your brain but it can also affect your heart and blood pressure and do serious harm to your liver. Your doctor will be able to help point you in the direction of the best available help for this.

Brain training

Does staying mentally fit keep your brain healthy in the same way that staying physically fit helps your body?

There's a multi-million-pound industry trying to suggest that it does and all sorts of games and program are available for use on home computers and most of the different gaming consoles.

The games work on the basis that regular use of computerized tests improves not only your score on those specific tests but also your cognitive function in general. Unfortunately, despite loads of research into the benefits of these games showing that the more people play them, the better they get at them, there is no evidence for that benefit being more generalized to other brain functions.

That doesn't mean it's not worth keeping the old grey matter active. A number of Alzheimer's charities advise that activities such as reading, writing for pleasure, learning new skills, hobbies, or foreign languages, and attending evening classes can help prevent dementia.

You only get one body and one brain. If you look after them, then the chances of developing a variety of disabling illnesses, including dementia, are greatly reduced.

Social activity

Those who don't get out much or mix with other people are known to be at greater risk of developing dementia than those who do. These social activities seem to keep thought processes in better shape and so protect against cognitive decline.

The simple message here is: don't sit indoors on your own with just the telly for company. Get out to lunch clubs, bingo, local faith-based groups, the cinema, or just round to see friends and relatives for a coffee and a chat.

10

Some final thoughts

Dementia is a condition whose signature symptoms are those of loss. Sufferers will lose their memory and their ability to relate to other people as they used to, and gradually they will become incapable of performing life's most simple tasks. Their personality can change too, leading us to feel that we have lost them as well.

I've dedicated this book to the memory of both my grandmother Hilda and my uncle George, who were both a big influence on my life as I grew up. Hilda spent hours on the floor with me, playing with soldiers and toy cars when I was a boy, and when I was at university would regularly bake the most fantastic lemon drizzle cakes for me and my housemates, to ensure that we at least had something other than pasta to eat. Uncle George was always happy to kick a ball around with me and my brother in his garden and, when we were teenagers, took us to the army camp where he worked so we could have a go at driving Chieftain battle tanks.

It was tragic for us as a family, and even more so for them, when dementia started to rob them of their memories and their ability to reason, to deal with money, and to carry out the day-to-day tasks that had always been second nature to them. As their conditions progressed, they first forgot our names and then failed to recognize us altogether. We watched as their worlds became so obviously bewildering to them. And we experienced the frustration of seemingly constant phone calls or knocks at the door to check and then recheck the answers to questions we'd given them many times already.

Losing someone to dementia is a bit like a bereavement. They may still be physically alive, but the part of them that was their emotional and psychological core, their soul even, seems dead. They are no longer the person we have always known them to be.

But they are still with us, and behind the confused and altered facade of a new persona is that person we have always known and loved. And just as they looked after us when we were younger, we owe it to them to do the same when they can no longer do it for themselves.

I hope that this short book has given an insight into the help that is available out there for people with dementia, and their carers, and that you will be more aware of how to access it. For although dementia is still incurable, there is a lot that can be done to ensure that its victims can have a reasonable quality of life. And there are techniques for connecting with people who may seem lost, because inside they are still the same mum, dad, husband, wife, grandparent, brother, or sister we have always known, and they need us to show them our love, however we can, more than ever.

Appendix A
The brain made easy

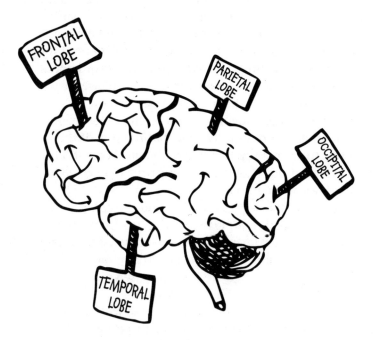

An adult brain is the most complex object in the entire universe, which is hard to believe when you look at it, because it resembles a giant blob of chewing gum. On average, it weighs 1.5 kilograms and has the consistency of either warm butter or tofu, depending on the eating habits of the brain surgeon who describes it to you. But it's a touch more complicated than either of these foods and can seem a bit baffling. So here's a basic, whistle-stop tour of some of its important structures and their functions.

Cerebral hemispheres
The brain is divided into two halves called cerebral hemispheres. Their outer layer of cells, called the cerebral cortex, looks grey, which is why the brain is often referred to as "grey matter". Each hemisphere is divided into four lobes which have different functions. These are called the frontal lobe, parietal lobe, temporal lobe, and occipital lobe.

Frontal lobe
This is the largest part of the whole brain. It makes us capable of higher functions such as planning and mental reasoning. It's a part of the brain that's far more developed in us than in any other animal species and is what has enabled us to conquer our environment, land on the moon, and even understand some of the more complicated laws of cricket. It is also involved in speech and movement, and is the main centre for our emotions.

Temporal lobe
This contains areas called the primary auditory cortex, which is involved in hearing; the hippocampus, which is important for turning short-term memories into long-term memories; and Wernicke's area, which allow us to understand language.

Parietal lobe
This area is important in movement and perception of sensations such as touch and pain. It also contains the primary sensory cortex, which helps us to analyse this

information when it comes into the brain from around the body. It also enables us to know which way is up.

Occipital lobe
A bit of a one-trick pony, this lobe is responsible for making sense of what we see and helps us to perceive shapes and colours.

Cerebral cortex
This is the layer of the brain where all the clever stuff goes on: memory, thought, language, and consciousness. It has different functions depending on which lobe it is in.

Brain stem
The cerebral hemispheres are perched on this stalk-like structure which connects the brain to the rest of the body through the spinal cord. It is the most primitive part of the brain, involved in controlling our most vital functions such as breathing and heartbeat. If this packs up, then so does everything else.

Cerebellum
This organ hangs off the back of the base of the cerebral hemispheres, looking uncannily like a piece of cauliflower. It's obviously far more complex than its doppelganger and is involved with posture, balance, and the coordination of movement. It is vital for fine-tuned movements such as picking up tiny objects in your fingers.

Ventricles
These are spaces within the brain tissue that are filled with cerebrospinal fluid.

Cerebrospinal fluid (CSF)

CSF circulates through the brain and around the spinal cord. It not only cushions the brain within the skull to protect it from damage during trauma but is also involved in removing the waste products produced during brain metabolism.

Brain cells

There are reckoned to be about 86 billion nerve cells, or neurones, in an adult brain, all working together to allow us to think, move, breathe, fall in love, watch our favourite soaps on TV, and understand this book. Enabling these and the many other functions of our brain to happen effectively requires more connections between these neurones per square centimetre of brain tissue than there are stars in our galaxy.

Brain cells pass messages between each other by conducting electricity. When the electrical signal reaches the end of one cell, the message is passed on to another, using chemicals called neurotransmitters. These pass across the gap between the cells (called a synapse), stick to receptors on the other side, which then trigger a further electrical signal to pass through the next cell, and so on. The transmitters are different in different parts of the brain. Some of the most commonly occurring and relevant to dementia are dopamine, glutamate, and, particularly where Alzheimer's disease is concerned, acetylcholine.

Memory

It's no exaggeration to say that a fully functioning memory is essential for normal human existence. In fact, without our memories, normal life is pretty much impossible. We are forever stuck in the moment that we are in and cannot learn from the past or plan for the future.

The way our memories work is still something of a scientific mystery, because it is an extremely complicated process involving a number of different parts of the brain. There are two different types of memory processes that occur: short-term and long-term memory.

Short-term memory

This is our working memory, which helps us remember things like telephone numbers. It has limited capacity and empties quickly to allow new memories to be stored. It's reckoned that it allows us to keep lists of five to nine items for around twenty to thirty seconds.

For a memory to stay in our heads beyond those first few seconds, it has to be transferred from short- to long-term memory where, theoretically, it could be stored for the rest of our lives.

Long-term memory

This has unlimited capacity and is divided into two main types, which psychologists have unfortunately given less than memorable names to:

- declarative memory: memory for facts such as phone numbers, meanings of words, general knowledge, events that have happened to you, sights, sounds, and smells from the past

- procedural memory: learning tasks and skills, such as riding a bike, wiring a plug, or tying your shoelaces.

All long-term memory needs three linked processes to happen for it to work effectively. Failure of one or all of these processes or a break in the links between them and the whole thing will fail. These processes are:

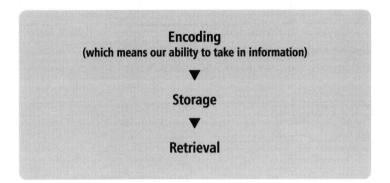

Encoding
(which means our ability to take in information)

▼

Storage

▼

Retrieval

A breakdown in these processes of encoding, storage, and retrieval can be seen in dementia.

 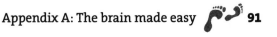

Appendix B
Sources of help and advice

This section provides contact details of a variety of state-run and charitable organizations that give advice about the physical and financial help and support available for people with dementia and their carers. It is by no means exhaustive but should provide some useful starting points.

United Kingdom

Age UK

Tavis House
1–6 Tavistock Square
London WC1H 9NA

Advice Line: 0800 169 6565

www.ageuk.org.uk

This new charity was formed by the amalgamation of Age Concern and Help the Aged. It provides advice and support for all older people.

Alzheimer's Society

Devon House
58 St Katharine's Way
London E1W 1LB

Helpline: 0300 222 11 22

www.alzheimers.org.uk

This is the leading charity for care and research into dementia in the UK. It provides excellent resources and information. The website has fact sheets on all aspects of dementia and its care and was one of many useful resources consulted when researching this book.

Benefit Enquiry Line

Warbreck House
Warbreck Hill Road
Blackpool FY2 0YE

0800 882 200

www.direct.gov.uk/benefits

National free advice on welfare benefits.

Carers Trust

32–36 Loman Street
London SE1 0EH

0844 800 4361

www.carers.org

Formed by the merger of Crossroads Care and The Princess Royal Trust for Carers, Carers Trust has schemes all over the UK offering practical support for carers.

Carers UK

20 Great Dover Street
London SE1 4LX

0808 808 7777

www.carersuk.org

Provides information for carers about how to access support.

Citizens Advice Bureau

www.citizensadvice.org.uk

Has offices all over the UK to provide advice and support on issues ranging from benefits to legal matters. Local offices can be found in the phone book and online.

NHS Direct

0845 4647

www.nhsdirect.nhs.uk

Offers 24-hour healthcare advice 365 days of the year on any matter.

Australia

Alzheimer's Australia

1 Frewin Place
Scullin
ACT 2614

02 6254 4233

National dementia helpline: 1800 100 500

www.fightdementia.org.au

Runs programmes all over the country offering support, education, counselling, and training for people with dementia, their carers, and health professionals.

Carers Australia

Unit 1
6 Napier Close
Deakin
ACT 2600

02 6122 9900

www.carersaustralia.com.au

A national organization which advocates for and supports carers and works with state and territory carers associations.

Government Benefits Advice

http://australia.gov.au/topics/benefits-payments-and-services

Website giving details of state welfare benefits.

National Welfare Rights Network

www.welfarerights.org.au

A national network of community legal centres which can advise and support people with their benefits applications and appeals.

Health Direct Australia

1800 022 222

A 24-hour helpline offering health advice from a registered nurse.

Canada

Alzheimer Society Canada

20 Eglinton Avenue West
16th Floor
Toronto
ON M4R 1K8

1 800 616 8816

www.alzheimer.ca

A national charity which funds research into dementia and offers advice and support for sufferers, professionals, and carers in English and French.

Service Canada

Service Canada
Canada Enquiry Centre
Ottawa ON K1A 0J9

1 800 622 6232

www.servicecanada.gc.ca/eng/lifeevents/caregiver.shtml

Gives advice about benefits, support, and options for carers.

Welfare Benefit Advice

1 800 622 6232

www.hrsdc.gc.ca/eng/disability_
issues/index.shtml

Government advice about benefit
entitlement.

New Zealand

Alzheimers New Zealand

4–12 Cruickshank Street
PO Box 14768
Kilbirnie
Wellington 6241

04 387 8264

www.alzheimers.org.nz

A national charity for those with
dementia and their carers which
has many local offices around the
country.

Carers New Zealand

PO Box 133
Mangonui
Far North 0442

09 406 0412

www.carers.net.nz

Provides information about benefits
and support for carers.

Healthline

0800 611 116

24-hour free telephone health advice.

USA

Alzheimer's Association

Alzheimer's Association National
Office
225 N. Michigan Avenue, Fl. 17
Chicago
IL 60601

24-hour helpline: 1 800 272 3900

www.alz.org

A national organization with local
chapters across the country involved
in care, support, and research.

Welfare Information

www.welfareinfo.org/payments

Welfare benefits in the USA will vary
from state to state. This is a useful
website to help get you started if you
want to apply.

Appendix C
Useful resources

In this book I have aimed to provide an accessible, up-to-date overview of the current medical thinking about the causes of and treatments for the symptoms of dementia. As a result I have summarized information on the subject from a wide range of books, websites, and medical journals, as well as drawing on my own experience.

In order to keep the text uncluttered, I have not listed them as I've gone along but would like to give particular mention to the following sources, which you may also find useful if you would like to read more about the subject.

The websites of the charities mentioned in Appendix B all provide excellent information about dementia, as do the following:

- www.nice.org.uk/TA217 (UK guidelines for best practice in the diagnosis and management of dementia)

- www.rcpsych.ac.uk (Royal College of Psychiatrists)

- www.netdoctor.co.uk and www.patient.co.uk (websites of medical advice for a range of conditions)

- www.nhs.uk (UK National Health Service website)

- Jonathan Foster, *Memory: A Very Short Introduction*, Oxford: Oxford University Press, 2009. This is a useful introduction to how memory is believed to work and what can go wrong when it becomes impaired and as we age.

Also currently available in the "First Steps" series:

First Steps out of Anxiety
Dr Kate Middleton

First Steps through Bereavement
Sue Mayfield

First Steps out of Depression
Sue Atkinson

First Steps out of Eating Disorders
Dr Kate Middleton
and Jane Smith

First Steps through the Menopause
Catherine Francis

First Steps out of Problem Drinking
John McMahon

First Steps out of Problem Gambling
Lisa Mills and Joanna Hughes

First Steps through Separation and Divorce
Penny Rich

First Steps out of Weight Problems
Catherine Francis

THE LONG TAIL

Chris Anderson is Editor-in-Chief of *Wired* magazine, a position he took in 2001. Since then he has led the magazine to five National Magazine Award nominations, winning the top prize for General Excellence in 2005, a year in which he was also named editor of the year by *AdAge* magazine. Previously he was at *The Economist, Nature,* and *Science* magazines. He has worked as a researcher at Los Alamos and served as research assistant to the Chief Scientist of the Department of Transportation. He lives in Northern California with his wife and four children. He can be reached at **www.thelongtail.com**.

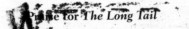

Praise for *The Long Tail*

Finalist for *The Financial Times* and Goldman Sachs Business Book of the Year 2006

'A brilliant and important book – as intelligent as it is e-entertaining.' **Robert Thomson, *The Times***

'*The Long Tail* . . . belongs on your shelf between *The Tipping Point* and *Freakonomics*, offering great insight into the next generation of internet revolution and opportunity.' **Reed Hastings, CEO Netflix**

'The Internet's long tail is driving the biggest transformation of media since the commercialization of television fifty years ago. Chris Anderson has done a masterful job of explaining the Long Tail and why it matters so much. Anyone who cares about media – indeed, anyone who cares about our society and where it's going – must read this book.' **Rob Glaser, CEO Real Networks**

'. . . a fascinating and hugely relevant study.' ***The Good Book Guide***

'Technology and the Internet are making the world a smaller and more connected place. *The Long Tail* is the first book to explain exactly how the ability to reach niche markets creates big opportunities.' **Terry Semel, CEO Yahoo!**